FAIRY LAND YOGA

ANTONIA PELLEGRINO-FREEMAN

Published in 2012 –
Copyright © Antonia Pellegrino-Freeman

First Edition

A CIP catalogue record for this title is available from the British Library.

ISBN-13:
978-1475181340

ISBN-10:
1475181345

Have you heard?

There is a place

To get to it we have to race,

This place is full of love and fun,

There's plenty of room for everyone!

The place I speak of is fairy land!

There's a fairy park and a fairy band,

A fairy tree house in a big old tree,

There's loads of space for you and me!

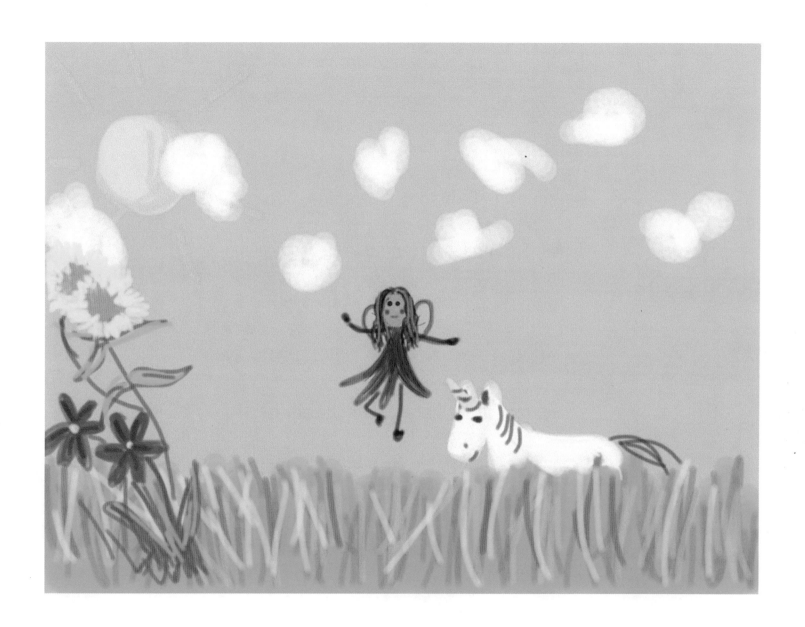

We have to wear some special clothes,

And rub some glitter on your nose.

The glitter helps us get there quick,

It is an age old fairy trick!

We need some wings so we can fly,

We'll pass the clouds and go so high.

We'll pass the mountains and the sea

I hope you can keep up with me!

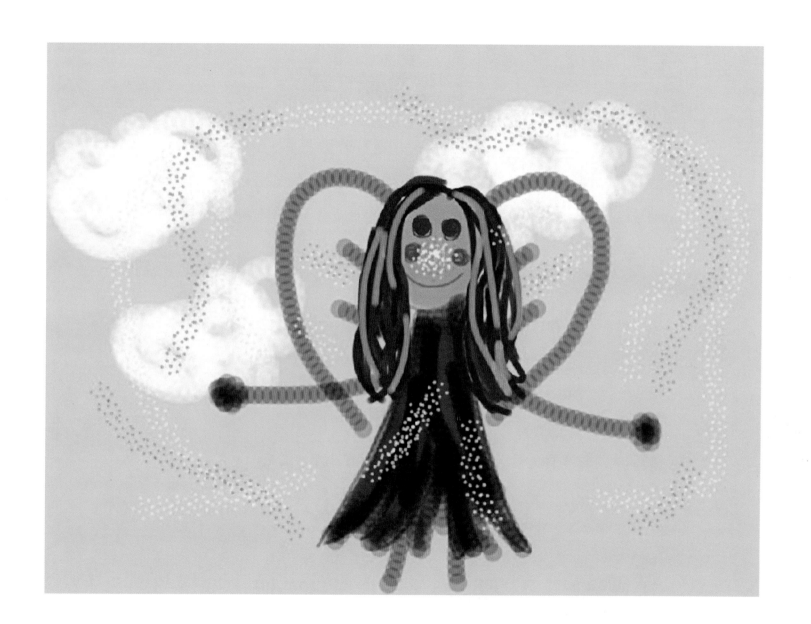

I promise you will love it here, Fairyland is very near!

Can you see the lights up there?

They shine and sparkle like a fair!

Now close your eyes, we have to land.

I'll keep you safe, just hold my hand!

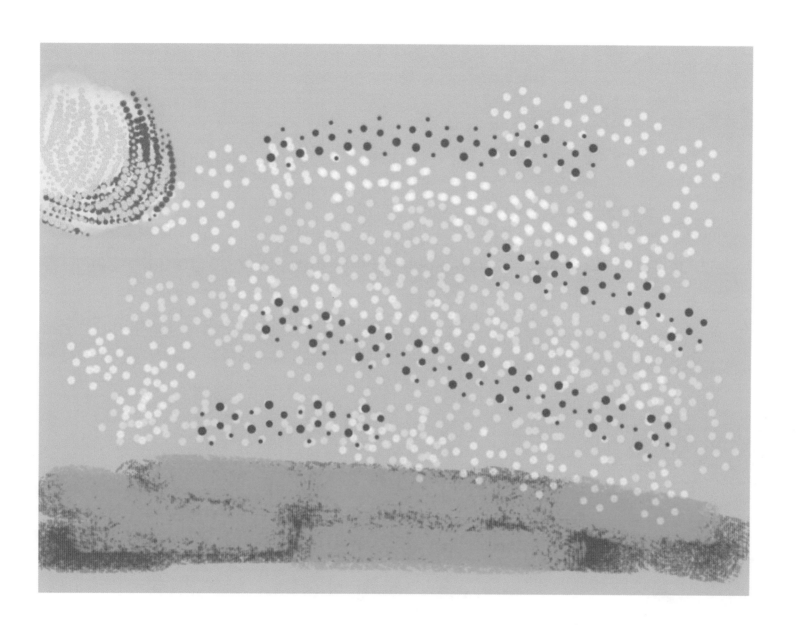

Wow we landed really well!

Can you sniff that scrumptious smell?

It smells like fruit trees; really sweet!

It must be the smell of fairy feet!

Fairies smell like summer fruits,

Their scent will fill the air!

The scent of orange from their wings and berries from their hair!

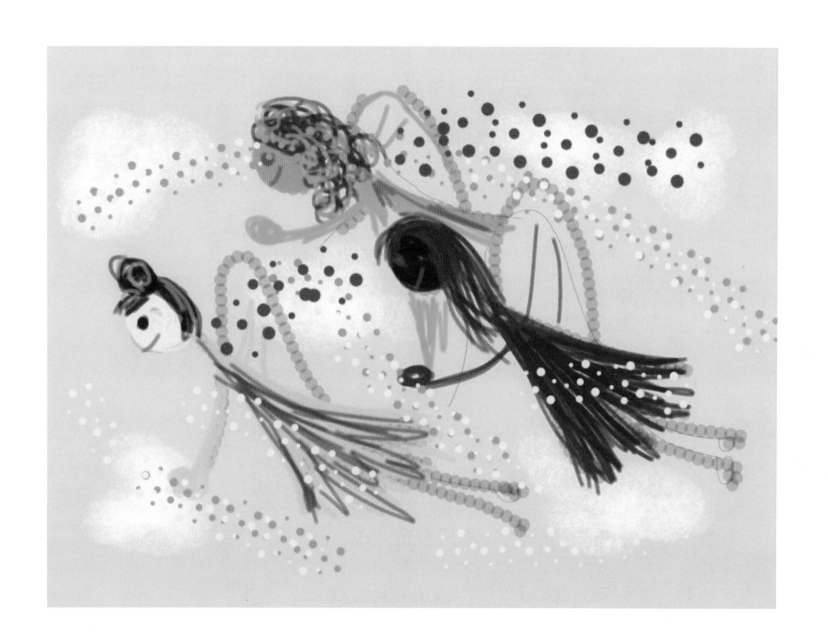

I've heard that fairies love to dance

And stretch their sparkly wings.

They love to balance twist and bend,

Whilst the princess fairy sings.

Let us join the fairy gang and learn to move and stand,

Fairy yoga on the carpet, grass and even sand

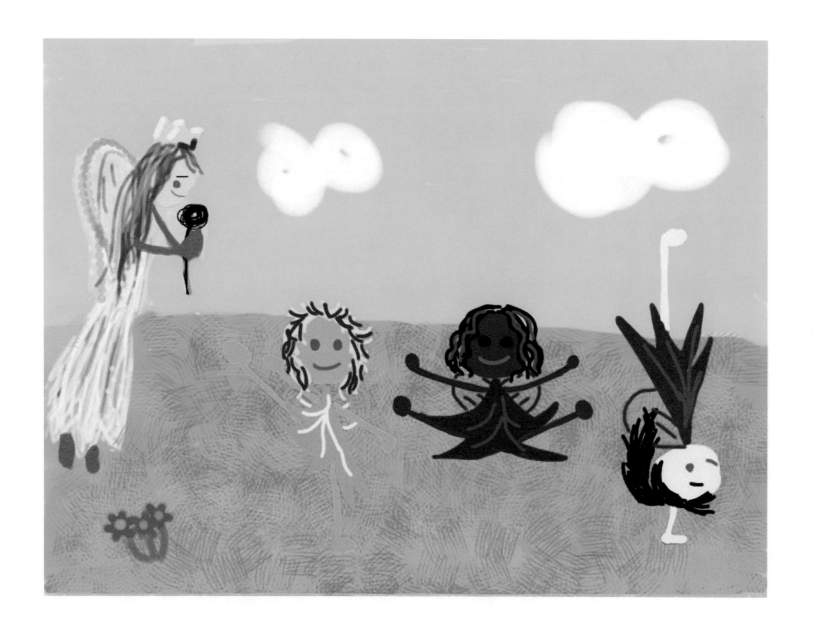

Fairies are so flexible and strong from top to toe

Some postures stretch us very high and some are really low.

We need to work both left and right, with equal energy,

Fairy yoga helps your body and your mind flow free!

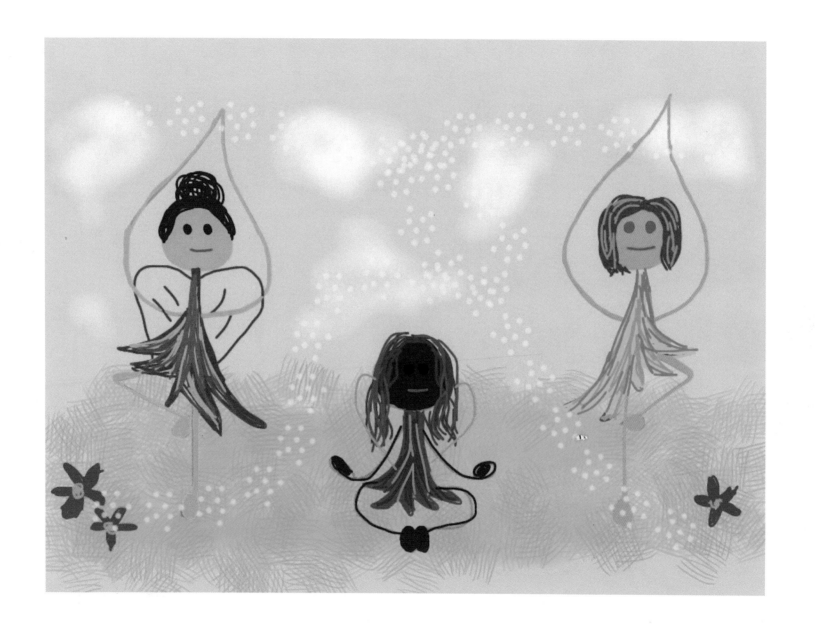

"We start by reaching way up high and drawing fairy wings.

Place your hands close by your heart!" The fairy princess sings.

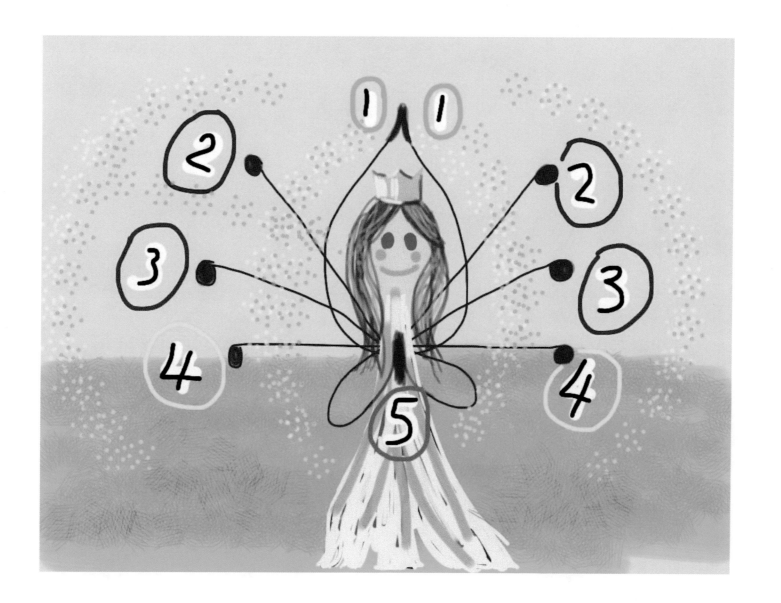

"Next we try to stretch our legs, walk your hands down to the floor.

Check that you have fairy tights, before we do some more.

Oh Wow! I see you normal clothes are now the fairy kind!

It's amazing all the things you can imagine with your mind!"

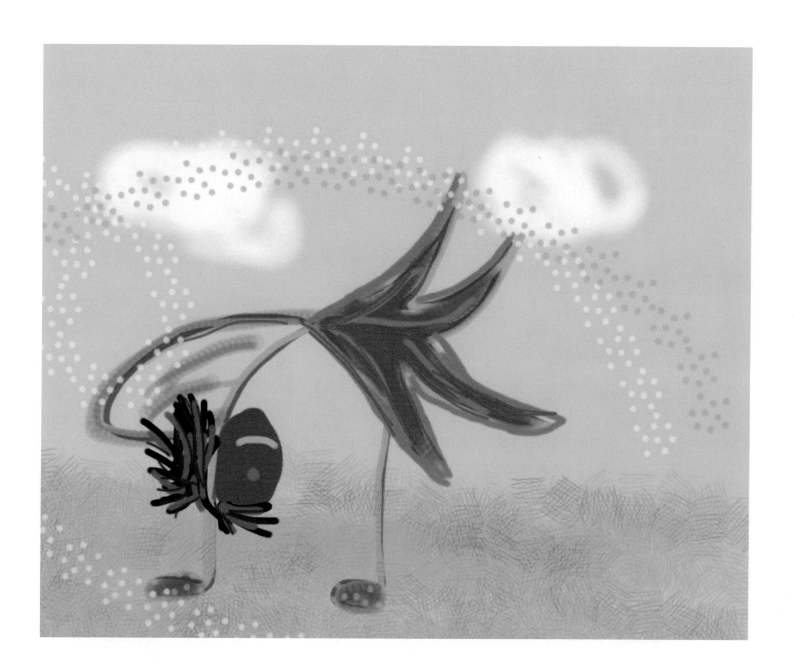

"Now we take a foot and place it way up on your thigh,

Pretend you are a swaying tree, with branches way up high!"

The fairies all applaud your stance, they cheer and clap with glee.

They all must think, you make a pretty awesome looking tree!

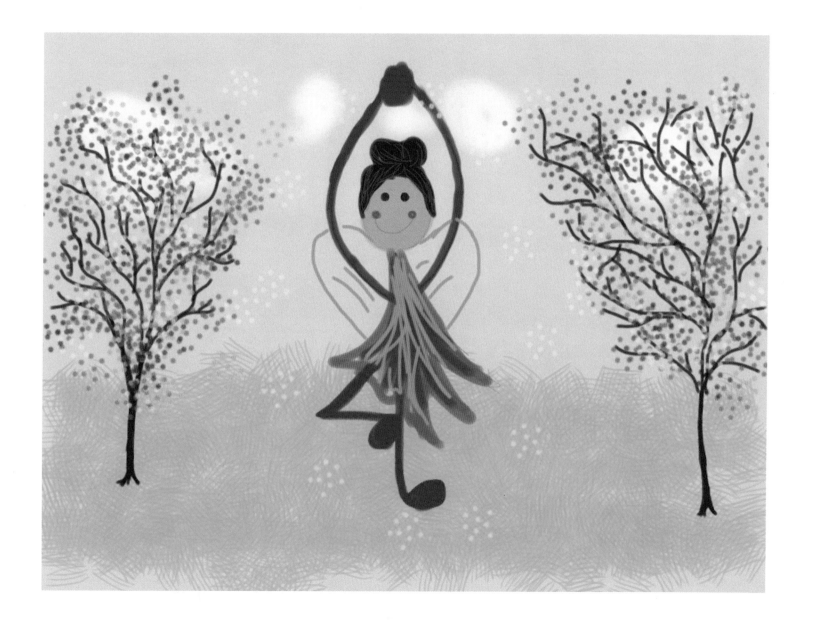

"Now we stretch our fairy skirts, way up into the sky,

This pose is called down facing dog , can you tell me why?

When puppies stretch, their legs go straight;

They stretch their tails and paws.

Now bend your knees, relax your back and come down to all fours."

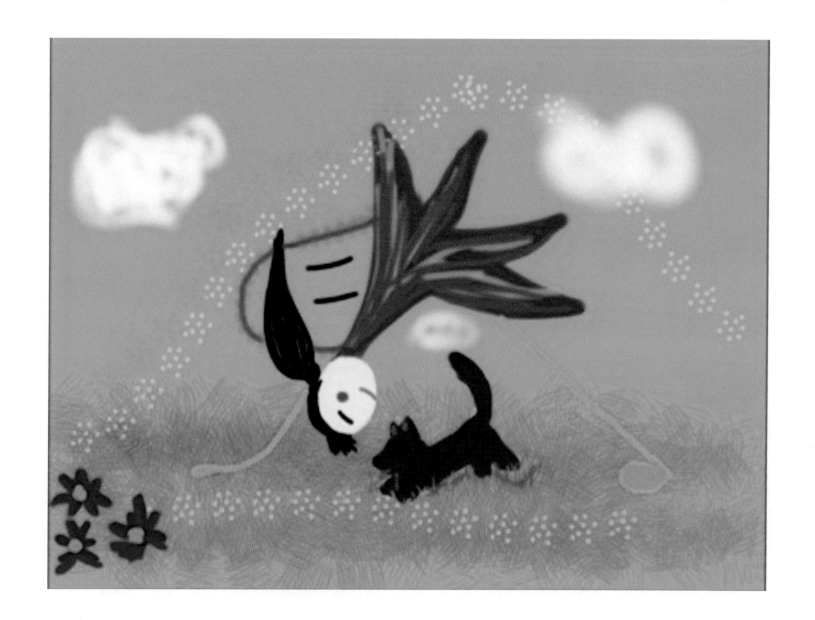

"Fairies love all animals, from unicorns to bats,

The next pose that we all shall do, is copying a cat.

So, on all fours we arch our backs, as far as you can go,

Make sure that you don't hold your breath,

Breathe deeply nice and slow!"

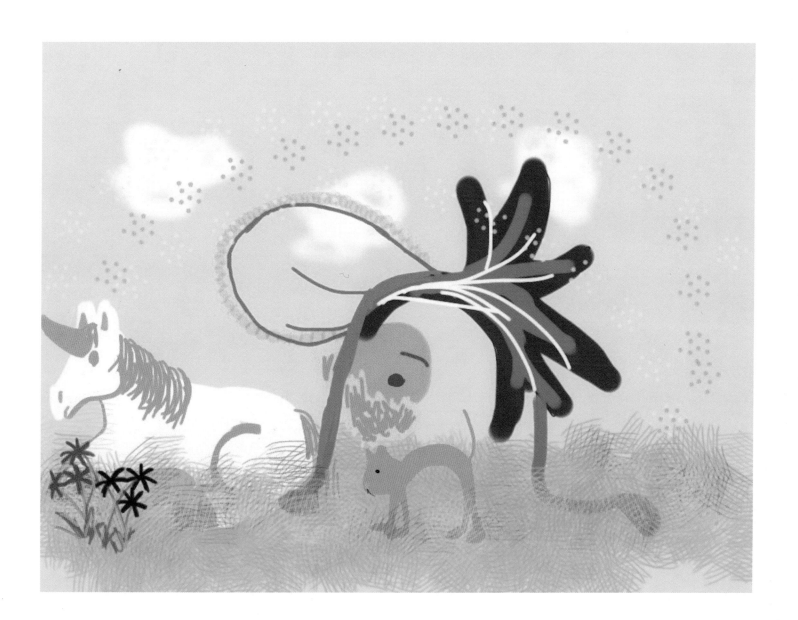

"Next we'll do the cobra, lying face down on the floor.

Stretch your body like a serpent, can you stretch a little more?

Lift your head whilst looking upwards, hands and elbows on the ground

You make a lovely cobra!

Can you make a 'hissy' sound?"

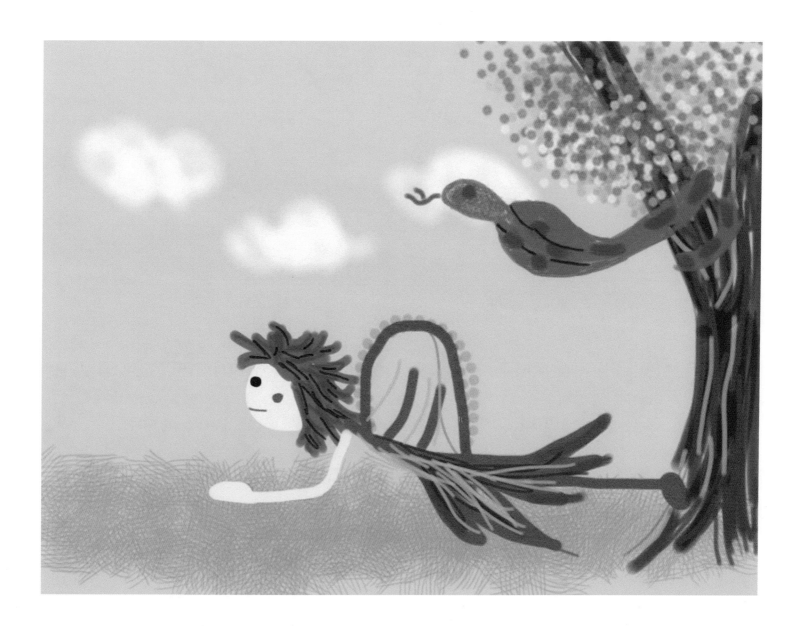

"As well as being gentle, Fairies can be very strong.

Let us stand in warrior pose" Goes the princess fairy song.

"Let's hold our special fairy wand and point it to the sky!

Bend one knee, the other straight, feel the strength build in your thigh!

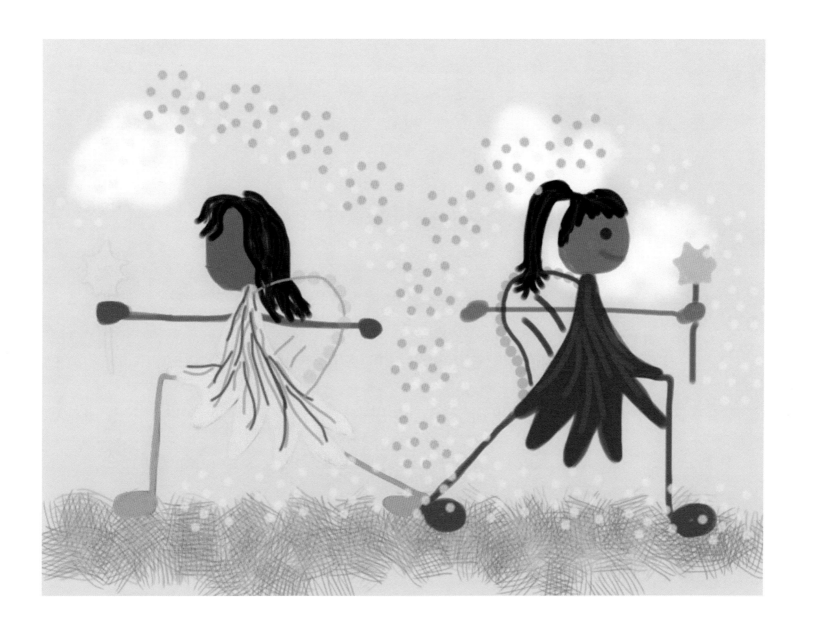

"There is a pose called triangle, all fairies love to do.

It stretches us from ponytails to sparkly fairy shoes.

Your feet apart, your legs stay straight, one hand is on your thigh,

Let's stretch our top arm to the sun. You can stretch up so high!"

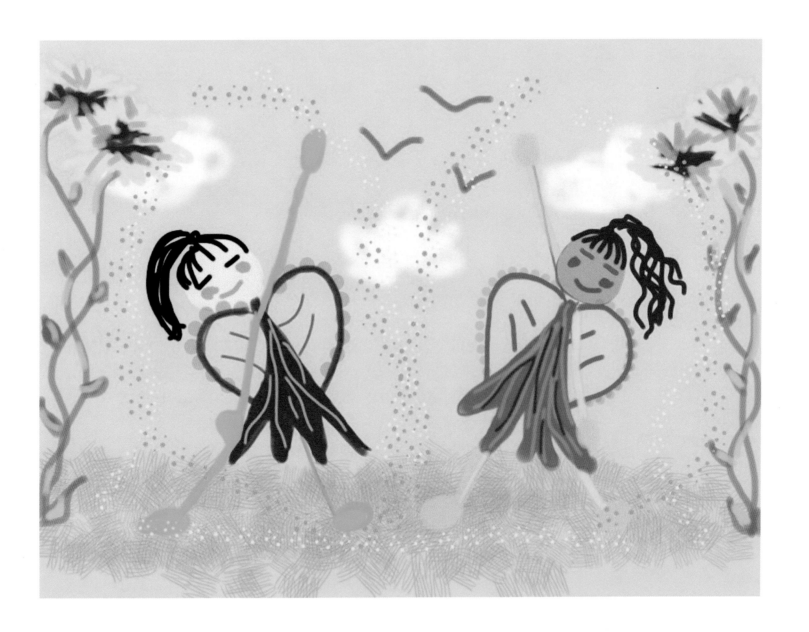

"Have you ever seen a star shoot right across the sky?

With silver sparkles make a wish and sing a lullaby.

We can make a wish come true, by standing like a star.

Lift one leg, bend to one side and balance where you are."

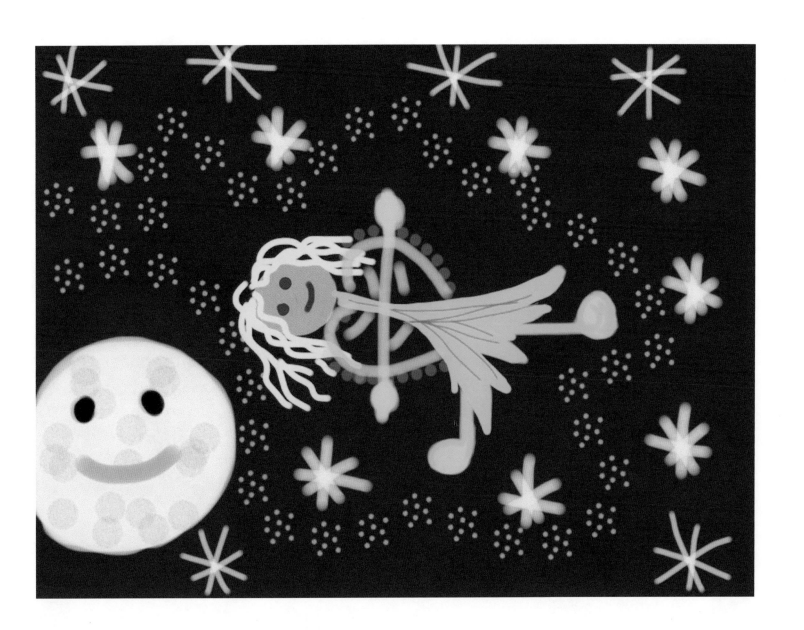

"You have been working very hard!"
The fairy princess smiles!

"You must have needed stretching, after flying all those miles!

Let's curl into a resting place, we call this 'the child's pose.'

Relax your mind, your arms and legs, your back and even nose.

Now close your eyes and count to ten, feel your body rest.

Fairy yoga helps us chill, it really is the best!"

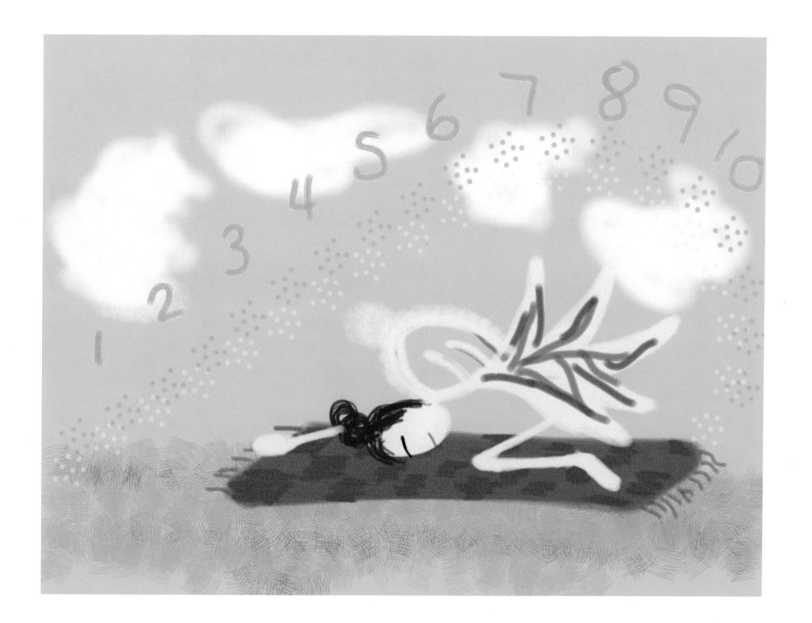

"Wiggle fairy fingers and wiggle fairy toes

Wiggle fairy bottoms and little sparkly nose

Wake your body up now. See the sights of fairy land.

Listen!

In the distance it's the lively fairy band!"

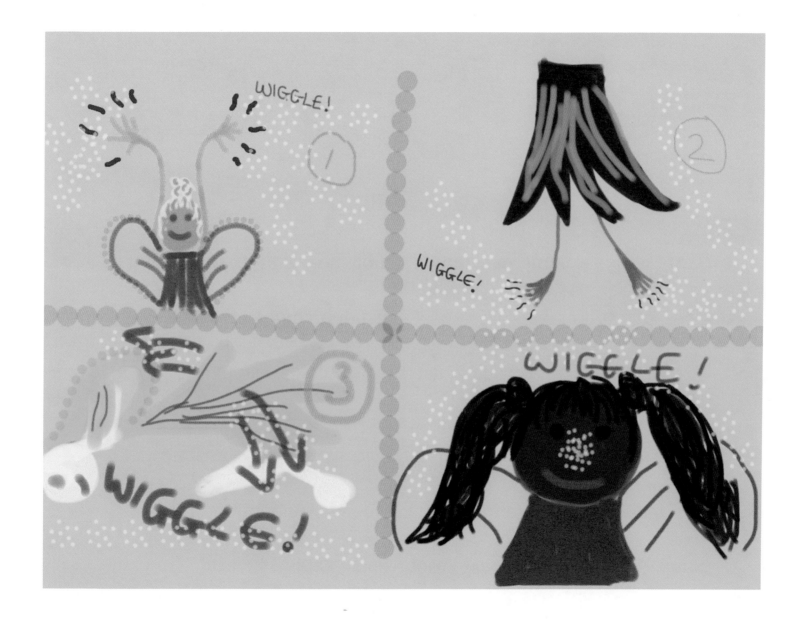

The fairy princess sings once more, when yoga time is done;

"Well done Fairy people, I hope that you had fun?

You came so far to be with us and practiced really
hard!

Fairy land is far from your back garden or your yard.

You must have past the moon and stars, the mountains and the sea?

We are so pleased that you could come, and now it's time for tea!"

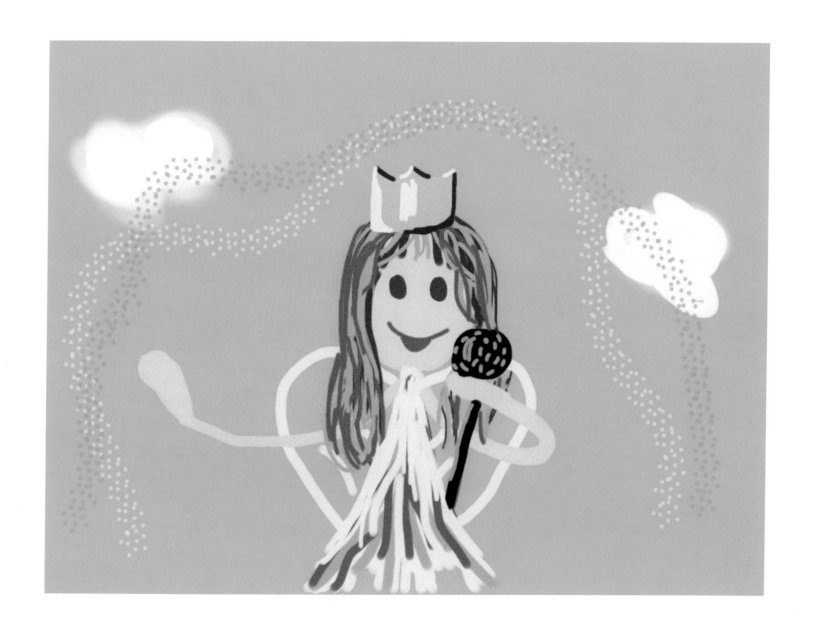

"Let's sit upon a blanket, with some fruit and fairy cake.

Fairies love to dance and sing, but also love to bake.

We'll drink from fairy glasses, made from petals, filled with dew

This special juice is fairy made from raindrops, just for you.

These special treats will help you, to safely return home,

They give you extra fairy power, wherever you may roam."

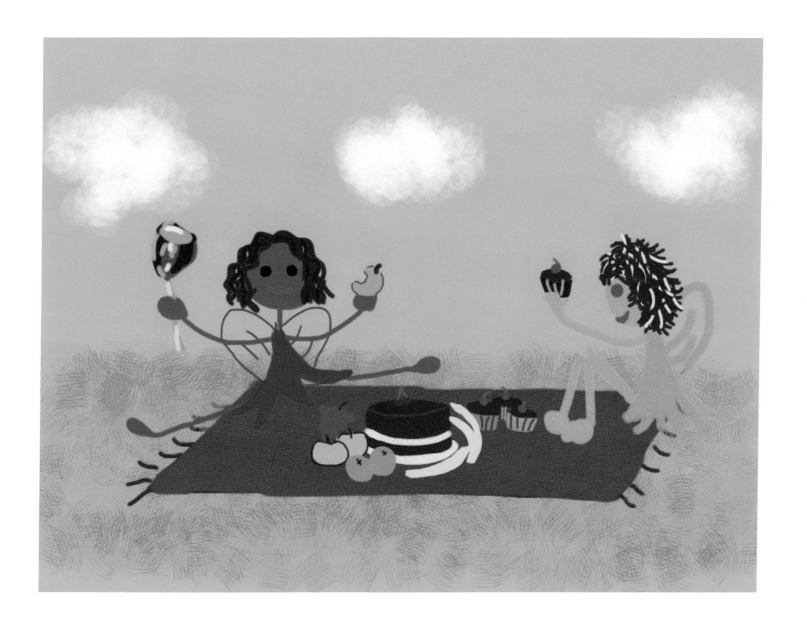

"When fairy tea is over, rub some glitter on your nose,

Sitting up cross legged, in this meditation pose.

With five deeps breaths close your eyes, imagine fairy land.

If you ever need to, you can practise where you stand!"

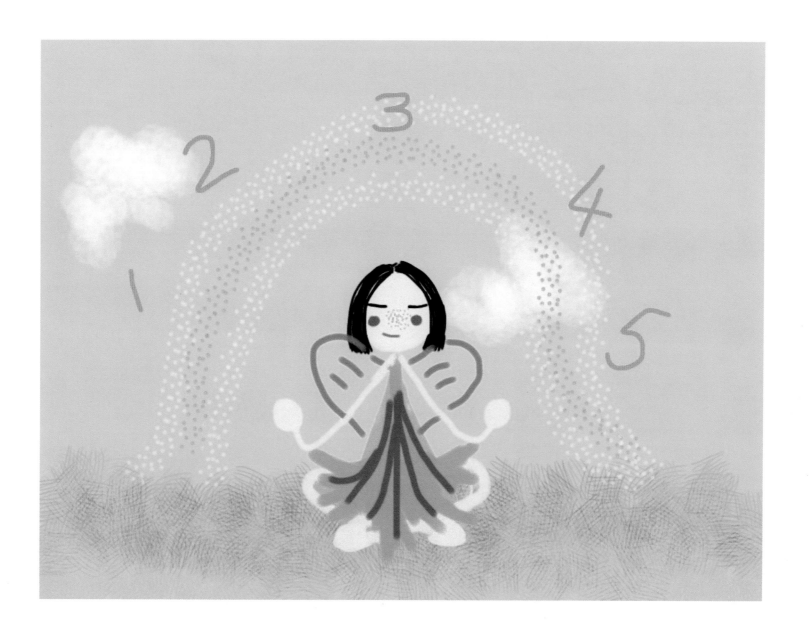

The fairies and the princess wave us off as we fly home

I'll keep you safe up in the air, you shan't fly back
alone!

You can always visit, the fairies wait in fairy land

Find a fun adventure. Turn the pages with your hand. xxxx

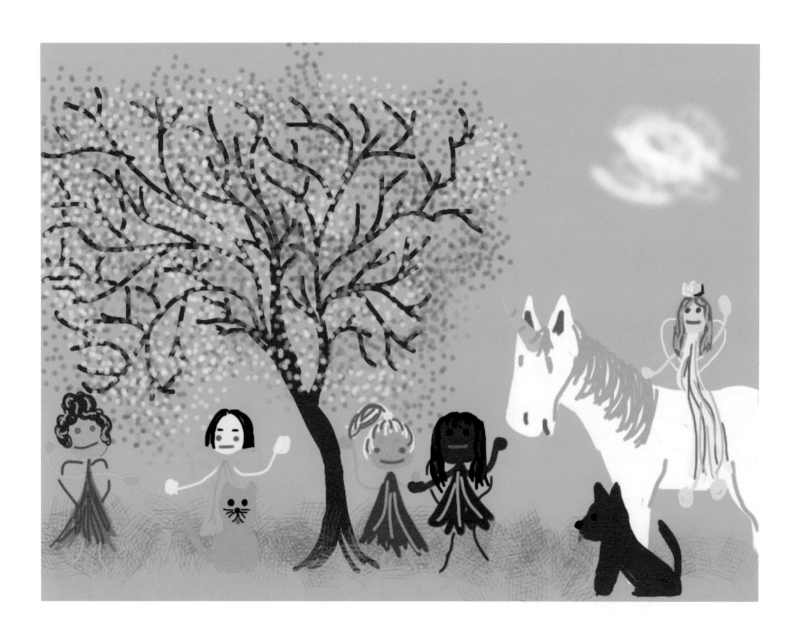

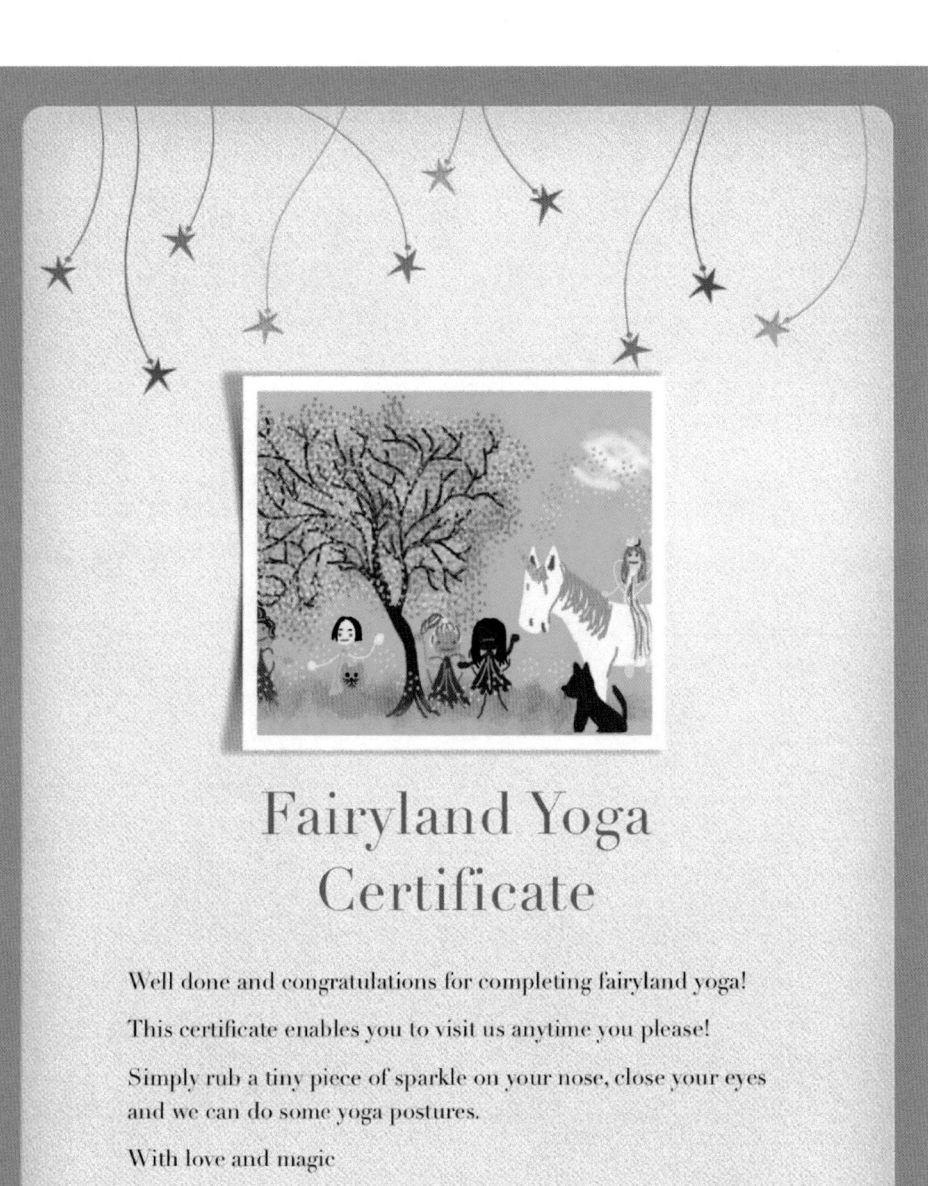

Fairyland Yoga Certificate

Well done and congratulations for completing fairyland yoga!

This certificate enables you to visit us anytime you please!

Simply rub a tiny piece of sparkle on your nose, close your eyes and we can do some yoga postures.

With love and magic

HRH Princess Fairy

Printed in Great Britain
by Amazon.co.uk, Ltd.,
Marston Gate.